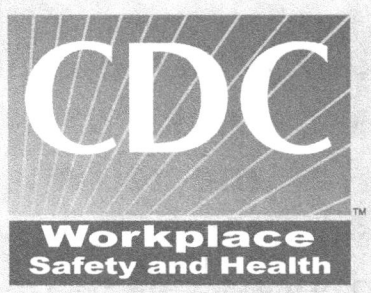

Formaldehyde Exposures During Brazilian Blowout Hair Smoothing Treatment at a Hair Salon – Ohio

Srinivas Durgam, MSPH, MSChE, CIH

Elena Page, MD, MPH

Health Hazard Evaluation Report
HETA 2011-0014-3147
November 2011

DEPARTMENT OF HEALTH AND HUMAN SERVICES
Centers for Disease Control and Prevention

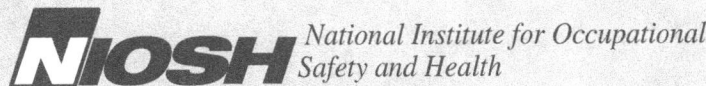

National Institute for Occupational Safety and Health

The employer shall post a copy of this report for a period of 30 calendar days at or near the workplace(s) of affected employees. The employer shall take steps to insure that the posted determinations are not altered, defaced, or covered by other material during such period. [37 FR 23640, November 7, 1972, as amended at 45 FR 2653, January 14, 1980].

CONTENTS

REPORT

APPENDIX

ACKNOWLEDGMENTS

ABBREVIATIONS

°F	Degrees Fahrenheit
ACGIH®	American Conference of Governmental Industrial Hygienists
AL	Action level
CAS	Chemical Abstract Service
CFR	Code of Federal Regulations
EPA	Environmental Protection Agency
FDA	Food and Drug Administration
GA	General area
HHE	Health hazard evaluation
HVAC	Heating, ventilating, and air-conditioning
MSDS	Material safety data sheet
NA	Not applicable
NAICS	North American Industry Classification System
NIOSH	National Institute for Occupational Safety and Health
OEL	Occupational exposure limit
OSHA	Occupational Safety and Health Administration
PBZ	Personal breathing zone
PPE	Personal protective equipment
PEL	Permissible exposure limit
ppm	Parts per million
REL	Recommended exposure limit
STEL	Short-term exposure limit
TLV®	Threshold limit value
TWA	Time-weighted average
WEEL™	Workplace environmental exposure level

HIGHLIGHTS OF THE NIOSH HEALTH HAZARD EVALUATION

The National Institute for Occupational Safety and Health (NIOSH) received an employer request for a health hazard evaluation at a hair salon in Ohio. The owner was concerned about employees' exposure to formaldehyde when performing hair smoothing treatments using Brazilian Blowout® hair products.

What NIOSH Did

- We visited the hair salon on December 13, 2010.

- We looked at work practices and conditions in the salon. We also looked at the processes used to apply the hair smoothing treatment.

- We took air samples for formaldehyde when no salon treatments were being done. We also took air samples when the hair smoothing treatment was being applied.

- We took bulk samples of three Brazilian Blowout hair products. We analyzed these for formaldehyde.

- We talked with employees about their work practices. We also asked them to fill out a survey about any symptoms they thought were related to their work.

What NIOSH Found

- Employee exposures to formaldehyde in air exceeded the NIOSH and American Conference of Governmental Industrial Hygienists' ceiling limits during the hair smoothing treatment.

- The Brazilian Blowout Acai Professional Smoothing Solution – Formaldehyde Free Smoothing Formula contained 11% formaldehyde, and the Brazilian Blowout Acai Professional Anti-Residue Shampoo contained 0.046% formaldehyde. The Brazilian Blowout Acai Deep Conditioning Masque contained 0.0013% formaldehyde.

- Employees reported no health symptoms during the hair smoothing treatment.

- Employees wore disposable latex gloves when applying the Brazilian Blowout Acai Professional Smoothing Solution – Formaldehyde Free Smoothing Formula to the hair.

What Managers Can Do

- Stop using the Brazilian Blowout Acai Professional Smoothing Solution – Formaldehyde Free Formula product.

- Follow the Occupational Safety and Health Administration formaldehyde standard if the salon continues to use this hair product.

HIGHLIGHTS OF THE NIOSH HEALTH HAZARD EVALUATION (CONTINUED)

- Tell employees about formaldehyde and its potential hazards to their health. Health effects can include cancer, irritation, and sensitization of the skin and respiratory system.

- Provide nitrile or butyl rubber gloves to reduce the risk of allergic reaction to natural latex.

What Employees Can Do

- Learn more about formaldehyde and how it can affect your health.

- Wear either nitrile or butyl rubber gloves when working with the Brazilian Blowout hair products.

SUMMARY

NIOSH investigators evaluated formaldehyde exposures from the Brazilian Blowout hair products in a hair salon. We found that employee exposures to formaldehyde exceeded the NIOSH and ACGIH ceiling limits during the treatment. The Brazilian Blowout Acai Professional Smoothing Solution – Formaldehyde Free Smoothing Formula contained 11% formaldehyde by weight. We recommended that the hair salon discontinue the use of this product.

In November 2010, NIOSH received an HHE request from the owner of a hair salon in Ohio. The request concerned employee exposure to formaldehyde when performing hair smoothing treatments using the Brazilian Blowout hair products.

We met with the employer and employee representatives on December 13, 2010. We looked at the hair treatment processes, work practices, and conditions at the salon. We collected air samples for formaldehyde at four locations in the salon when no treatment was being conducted. We then collected air samples on a hairstylist performing the Brazilian Blowout treatment and another hairstylist working in the salon. We collected bulk samples of the Brazilian Blowout Acai Professional Smoothing Solution – Formaldehyde Free Smoothing Formula, the Brazilian Blowout Acai Professional Anti-Residue Shampoo, and the Brazilian Blowout Acai Deep Conditioning Masque from their original containers. We also talked with employees about their work practices and asked them to complete a survey about their symptoms.

The PBZ air sample results for formaldehyde exceeded the NIOSH ceiling limit of 0.1 ppm and the ACGIH ceiling limit of 0.3 ppm but did not exceed the OSHA STEL of 2 ppm. Bulk sample analyses indicated that the Brazilian Blowout Acai Professional Smoothing Solution – Formaldehyde Free Smoothing Formula contained 11% formaldehyde, and the Brazilian Blowout Acai Professional Anti-Residue Shampoo contained 0.046% formaldehyde. The Brazilian Blowout Acai Deep Conditioning Masque contained 0.0013% formaldehyde. All three employees present in the salon on the day of our evaluation completed the survey. None of these employees reported symptoms while the treatment was being applied, but one did report throat irritation when applying the product in the past.

We recommended that the hair salon discontinue the use of the Brazilian Blowout Acai Professional Smoothing Solution – Formaldehyde Free Formula product. If the salon continues to use this product, it should follow the requirements listed in the OSHA formaldehyde standard. The employer should also discuss specific health hazards associated with formaldehyde with its employees. These health hazards include cancer, irritation, and sensitization of the skin and respiratory system. Employees should wear nitrile or butyl rubber gloves to reduce the risk of an allergic reaction to latex.

Keywords: NAICS 812112 (Beauty Salons), formaldehyde (CAS number 50-00-0), hair salon, Brazilian Blowout, smoothing, hair treatment, acai

This page left intentionally blank

INTRODUCTION

In November 2010, NIOSH received an HHE request from the owner of a hair salon in Ohio. The request concerned hairstylists' exposure to formaldehyde when performing hair smoothing treatments with the Brazilian Blowout hair product. We met with the employer and employee representatives on December 13, 2010. We conducted this evaluation on a day when the hair salon was closed. One of the hairstylists was planning to receive the hair smoothing treatment, and we used this opportunity to conduct the evaluation. Therefore, the two stylists and the salon owner were present during the evaluation. The results of this evaluation were shared with the employer in an interim letter dated May 16, 2011.

Background

In early 2010 the Oregon Health Sciences University became aware that employees of a hair salon in Portland, Oregon, were experiencing health symptoms such as difficulty breathing, nosebleeds, and eye irritation when using a popular hair smoothing product manufactured by Brazilian Blowout. Responding to an Oregon Health Sciences University request, Oregon OSHA analyzed a bulk sample of the "Formaldehyde Free" labeled version of the hair smoothing product and found that it contained 8.5% formaldehyde. This discovery led to an enforcement initiative by Oregon OSHA and the collection of additional bulk samples and air monitoring in Oregon hair salons. On the basis of these results, Oregon OSHA issued an alert advising salons to take necessary precautions including training workers and conducting air monitoring to ensure workers were not exposed to formaldehyde levels above the OSHA PEL of 0.75 ppm [Oregon OSHA 2010a,b].

Since the alert was issued by Oregon OSHA (October 29, 2010), federal OSHA, several state OSHA programs, Health Canada, and the U.S. FDA have published alerts and advisories on the use of hair smoothing products that contain or release formaldehyde. Specifically identified in these reports is the Brazilian Blowout hair product line. These alerts and advisories cite a number of studies where air sampling measured formaldehyde from hair smoothing products that were labeled as "formaldehyde-free" [California OSHA 2010; Consumer Federation of America 2011; FDA 2011; Health Canada 2011; OSHA 2011].

News reports of health concerns and the presence of formaldehyde in keratin-based hair smoothing products such as Brazilian Blowout were reported as early as 2007 [Fischer 2007; Hayt 2007]. The media used these alerts and advisories to highlight the use and safety of such products [Pristin 2010; Rabin 2010; Anderson 2011; Athavaley 2011a,b; Associated Press 2011].

Process Description

The hair salon was located in a converted single family house. The salon had a reception area, hair treatment room, hair wash/dry room, and a dispensary room that also served as a break area for hairstylists. The dispensary room contained various hair products including hair colors, shampoos, and other treatment products that were stored in their original containers. The Brazilian Blowout Acai Professional Smoothing Solution – Formaldehyde Free Smoothing Formula was dispensed into smaller containers in this room before being applied to a client's hair. The hair salon had a thermostatically-controlled residential HVAC system in the basement. The HVAC system used 1-inch thick pleated fiberglass air filters, and the supply air was delivered through floor vents.

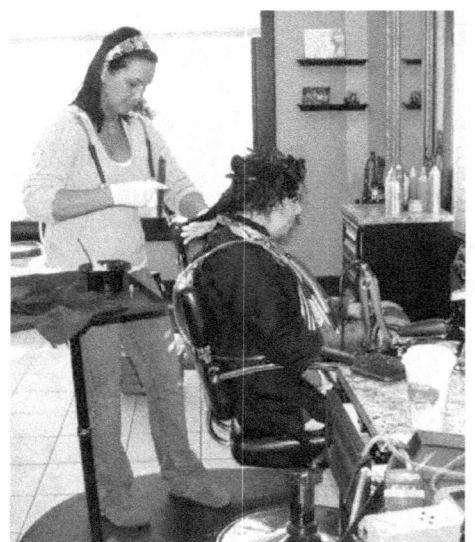

Figure 1. Formaldehyde air sampling conducted while a hairstylist applies Brazilian Blowout smoothing solution to the hair.

This hair salon offered a variety of hair treatments including the Brazilian Blowout, one of many commercially available keratin-based hair smoothing treatments. The Brazilian Blowout treatment process has six steps:

- Hair was washed with the Brazilian Blowout Acai Professional Anti-Residue Shampoo in the hair wash/dry room.

- The hairstylist used a brush to apply the Brazilian Blowout Acai Professional Smoothing Solution – Formaldehyde Free Smoothing Formula to all parts of the wet hair in a systematic fashion in the hair treatment room. The hairstylist wore disposable latex gloves during this stage of the treatment only (Figure 1).

- Hair was then brushed and blow dried with an Artizen® 3300 5kV Ionic hair dryer that was set at the highest heat setting.

- A flat iron set at 450°F was used four to five times on each section of the hair (Figure 2).

- The Brazilian Blowout Acai Deep Conditioning Masque was then applied to the dried hair and rinsed off with water in the hair wash/dry room.

- Hair was again blow dried with the same hair dryer in the hair treatment room.

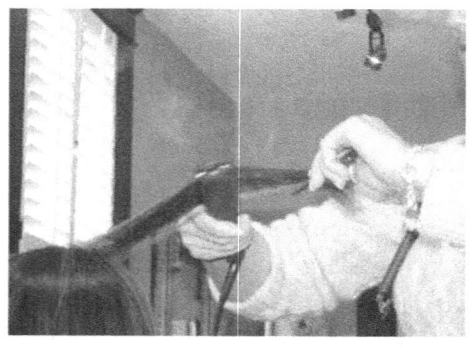

Figure 2. Flat ironing a section of hair – visible smoke was observed during this task.

ASSESSMENT

During the visit we discussed the HHE request with the employer, the hairstylist conducting the Brazilian Blowout treatment, and the hairstylist receiving the treatment. We observed work processes, practices, and workplace conditions and spoke with employees. We reviewed the MSDS (revision date October 26, 2010) for the Brazilian Blowout Professional Smoothing Solution that the employer indicated was for the Brazilian Blowout Acai Professional Smoothing Solution – Formaldehyde Free Smoothing Formula and the treatment summary sheet. MSDSs were not available for the Brazilian Blowout Acai Professional Anti-Residue Shampoo nor for the Brazilian Blowout Acai Deep Conditioning Masque. We also administered questionnaires to employees to assess work-related health symptoms.

To evaluate the background levels of formaldehyde in the hair salon, we collected GA air samples for formaldehyde at four locations throughout the hair salon from 0840–1240 hours when no treatments were being conducted. During the Brazilian Blowout treatment, we collected PBZ air samples on the hairstylist who performed each of the six tasks of the treatment as well as short-term samples during specific times within each of the six tasks. We also collected a PBZ air sample for formaldehyde on the other hairstylist working in the salon. GA air samples were also collected at the same four locations used for background samples in the hair salon.

Formaldehyde air samples were collected according to NIOSH Method 2016 using silica gel tubes coated with 2,4-dinitrophenyl hyrdrazine (Part No. 226-210, SKC Inc., Eighty Four, Pennsylvania) and air sampling pumps that were calibrated before and after use at flow rates of either 50 or 200 cubic centimeters per minute [NIOSH 2011]. These samples were analyzed for formaldehyde and other aldehydes including acetaldehyde, benzaldehyde, and butyraldehyde, as well as acetone and methyl ethyl ketone. The analysis was conducted by high performance liquid chromatography according to EPA Method TO-11 [EPA 2011].

We collected bulk samples of the Brazilian Blowout Acai Professional Smoothing Solution – Formaldehyde Free Smoothing Formula, the Brazilian Blowout Acai Professional Anti-Residue Shampoo, and the Brazilian Blowout Acai Deep Conditioning Masque from their original containers. These bulk samples were analyzed by high performance liquid chromatography using an ultraviolet detector as described in the Oregon OSHA report [Oregon OSHA 2010a].

RESULTS

Results of the task-based and short-term PBZ air samples collected on the hairstylist performing the Brazilian Blowout treatments are presented in Table 1. The formaldehyde concentrations for the task-based air samples ranged from 0.018–1.1 ppm. The short-term sample concentrations ranged from 0.018–1.3 ppm. We measured the highest formaldehyde concentration during product application (both the task-based and the short-term air samples), followed by blow drying and flat ironing. All but two of the short-term air samples exceeded the NIOSH ceiling limit of 0.1 ppm, and four samples exceeded the ACGIH ceiling limit of 0.3 ppm. None of the PBZ samples exceeded the OSHA STEL of 2 ppm.

Table 1. PBZ air sampling results for formaldehyde taken on a hairstylist performing the Brazilian Blowout smoothing treatment

Task	Task-based		Short-term	
	Sampling Time (minutes)	Concentration (ppm)	Sampling Time (minutes)	Concentration (ppm)
Hair Washing	10	0.018	9	0.018
Product Application	33	1.1	16	0.36
			18	1.3
Blow Drying Post Application	20	0.78	19	0.90
Flat Ironing	20	0.46	16	0.36
Masque Application and Hair Wash	11	0.25*	15	0.24
Blow Drying Post Washing	18	0.14	19	0.12

*Backup section collected > 10% of the front section, so concentration may be underestimated.

We collected a PBZ sample on the other hairstylist in the salon, and the formaldehyde concentration was 0.10 ppm for a sampling period of 112 minutes (the duration of the Brazilian Blowout treatment). This hairstylist was cutting hair and conducting other salon tasks and was positioned approximately 6 feet from where the Brazilian Blowout treatment was being performed.

Results of the GA air sampling for formaldehyde are presented in Table 2. When no treatment was performed, the GA air concentrations of formaldehyde ranged from 0.0044–0.025 ppm. The highest formaldehyde concentration (0.025 ppm) was measured in the dispensary and may be the result of pouring the Brazilian Blowout Acai Professional Smoothing Solution – Formaldehyde Free Smoothing Formula from the manufacturer's bottle into a small dish before starting the treatment. When

RESULTS
(CONTINUED)

the Brazilian Blowout treatment was performed, the GA air concentrations of formaldehyde ranged from 0.057–0.11 ppm, with the highest formaldehyde concentration measured in the hair treatment room.

Table 2. GA air sampling results for formaldehyde

Area	No Treatment		Brazilian Blowout Treatment	
	Sampling Time (minutes)	Concentration (ppm)	Sampling Time (minutes)	Concentration (ppm)
Reception Desk	238	0.0069*	145	0.062
Hair Treatment Room	244	0.0087	144	0.11
Hair Wash/Dry Room	247	0.0044	143	0.057
Dispensary	390	0.025	NA	NA

*Backup section collected > 10% of the front section, so concentration may be underestimated.

Acetone, methyl ethyl ketone, and other aldehydes were not detected in most of the PBZ and GA air samples. The highest air concentrations (acetaldehyde, acetone, benzaldehyde, valeraldehyde) were observed during the flat ironing task of the treatment but were all less than 1% of the applicable short-term OELs.

The Brazilian Blowout Acai Professional Smoothing Solution – Formaldehyde Free Smoothing Formula contained 11% formaldehyde by weight, and the Brazilian Blowout Acai Professional Anti-Residue Shampoo contained 0.046% formaldehyde by weight. The Brazilian Blowout Acai Deep Conditioning Masque contained 0.0013% formaldehyde by weight, a concentration above the limit of detection but below the limit of quantitation of 0.0060% of our analytical method; hence this reported concentration has uncertainty associated with it.

The three employees present in the salon filled out our questionnaire. One applied the treatment, one received the treatment, and one was performing other duties. No one reported symptoms while the treatment was applied, but one employee reported throat irritation when applying the product in the past. All reported using latex gloves when applying the treatment.

DISCUSSION

Employees in hair salons are exposed to a variety of chemicals that are constituents of the products used in the trade [Labreche et al. 2003; Mendes et al. 2011]. Some of these ingredients, including formaldehyde, have been found to be carcinogenic by the International Agency for Research on Cancer [Labreche et al. 2003]. Formaldehyde (CAS number 50-0-0) is a colorless gas at room temperature and is known and marketed in products under various names, including methanal, methylene oxide, formalin, and methylene glycol [NIST 2011]. (Note: the CAS number is a unique identifier assigned to chemicals.) Formaldehyde in a solution of water containing alcohol stabilizer is referred to as formalin and has the same CAS number of 50-0-0. However, formaldehyde when dissolved in water forms a diol called methylene glycol or methane diol, which has a different CAS number of 463-57-0. Formaldehyde gas and the methylene glycol solution exist in a dynamic and reversible equilibrium, and therefore, the aqueous solution is capable of releasing formaldehyde gas [Winkelman et al. 2002; Oregon OSHA 2010a; Consumer Federation of American 2011]. An Oregon OSHA report concluded that for the purposes of worker protection it is appropriate to refer to both the hydrated and the non-hydrated formaldehyde as formaldehyde [Oregon OSHA 2010a]. In addition, the OSHA formaldehyde standard applies to all occupational exposures to formaldehyde (i.e , formaldehyde gas) its solutions, and other materials that release formaldehyde [29 CFR 1910.1048].

In this evaluation we intended to measure employee exposures during each hair treatment task while simultaneously collecting shorter-term (approximately 15-minute) air samples for comparison with applicable OELs. However, during our evaluation we learned that the duration of each hair treatment task depended on factors such as the client's hair length and the hairstylist's skill level. For this evaluation the duration of all of the hair treatment tasks (except product application) was short, resulting in similar sampling times for both the task and short-term air samples. Because in other hair treatments this may not necessarily be the case, we believe it would be helpful to continue collecting both task-based and short-term air samples.

Our PBZ air sampling results showed that the hairstylist using the Brazilian Blowout Acai Professional Smoothing Solution – Formaldehyde Free Smoothing Formula was exposed to formaldehyde air concentrations that exceeded the NIOSH ceiling limit during all Brazilian Blowout treatment tasks except

DISCUSSION
(CONTINUED)

the initial hair wash. The ACGIH ceiling limit was exceeded during the product application, blow drying post application, and flat ironing tasks of the treatment. None of the reported formaldehyde concentrations exceeded the OSHA PEL or OSHA STEL. These results are consistent with the Oregon OSHA findings from its evaluation of seven salons that used the same "formaldehyde free" product [Oregon OSHA 2010a]. However, federal OSHA test results have shown that formaldehyde levels in a hair salon have exceeded the OSHA OELs when hairstylists use the Brazilian Blowout Acai Professional Smoothing Solution – Formaldehyde Free Smoothing Formula [OSHA 2011]. OSHA provided recommendations to limit worker exposures, including using air ventilation systems to keep formaldehyde levels below OSHA's exposure limits, performing regular maintenance on these systems to ensure proper operation, and using lower heat settings on flat irons and blow dryers [OSHA 2011]. Use of local exhaust ventilation in hair salons has been documented to reduce exposure levels to contaminants when compared to salons with no local exhaust ventilation [Hollund and Moen 1998].

The GA air sample results suggest that hairstylists and other salon employees (especially those working near the treatment) can be exposed to formaldehyde air concentrations during the Brazilian Blowout treatment above background levels. Further sampling is needed to characterize their full-shift personal exposures to formaldehyde.

We found that the Brazilian Blowout Acai Professional Smoothing Solution – Formaldehyde Free Smoothing Formula contained 11% formaldehyde by weight, which is similar to the average formaldehyde content of 8.8% reported by Oregon OSHA for the same "formaldehyde free" product [Oregon OSHA 2010a]. We also found that the Brazilian Blowout Acai Professional Anti-Residue Shampoo contained 0.046% formaldehyde, which is similar to the 0.05% average formaldehyde content reported by Oregon OSHA for this same shampoo [Oregon OSHA 2010a].

Because we found formaldehyde air concentrations greater than 0.1 ppm, and the Brazilian Blowout Acai Professional Smoothing Solution – Formaldehyde Free Smoothing Formula contained formaldehyde at greater than 0.1%, the hazard communication requirements of the OSHA formaldehyde standard are applicable [29 CFR 1910.1048(m)]. This standard requires employers to discuss specific health hazards with their employees including

Discussion (continued)

cancer, irritation, and sensitization of the skin and respiratory system. The standard also requires a written hazard communication program that includes requirements for MSDSs and employee training.

The OSHA formaldehyde standard requires that manufacturers provide their downstream users (such as hairstylists) with accurate MSDSs that address health hazards associated with exposure to formaldehyde. In addition, manufacturers are required to modify their labels to indicate the presence of formaldehyde in their product. If the product is capable of releasing formaldehyde at levels exceeding 0.5 ppm over an 8-hour work shift, the label shall contain the words "Potential Cancer Hazard."

The MSDS provided by the manufacturer to the hair salon for the product it uses (the Brazilian Blowout Acai Professional Smoothing Solution – Formaldehyde Free Smoothing Formula) stated that it contained less than 5% methylene glycol. However, this MSDS did not state specifically that it was for the Formaldehyde Free Smoothing Formula. We contacted the product manufacturer directly to inquire whether the Brazilian Blowout Professional Smoothing Solution MSDS was for the "Formaldehyde Free Smoothing Formula" used by the hair salon during our evaluation and to request MSDSs for the Brazilian Blowout Acai Professional Anti-Residue Shampoo and Brazilian Blowout Acai Deep Conditioning Masque. We received MSDSs for all three products but none of the product names on the MSDSs were the same as the product labels. However, we were assured by the manufacturer that they were correct [Dalva 2011]. In addition, the "Formaldehyde Free" portion of the product label has been removed. The MSDSs for the Brazilian Blowout Acai Professional Anti-Residue Shampoo and Brazilian Blowout Acai Deep Conditioning Masque listed no hazardous components.

The hair salon should be aware that salon product MSDSs may not list formaldehyde as being present or may list formaldehyde under other names such as methylene glycol, methane diol, formalin, methylene oxide, paraform, formic aldehyde, methanal, oxomethane, oxymethylene, or CAS Numbers 50-00-0 and 463-57-0.

CONCLUSIONS

The hairstylist performing hair smoothing treatment with the Brazilian Blowout Acai Professional Smoothing Solution – Formaldehyde Free Formula product was exposed to formaldehyde air concentrations that exceed the NIOSH and ACGIH ceiling limits.

RECOMMENDATIONS

On the basis of our findings, we recommend the actions listed below to create a more healthful workplace. We encourage the hair salon to use a labor-management health and safety committee or working group to discuss the recommendations in this report and develop an action plan. Those involved in the work can best set priorities and assess the feasibility of our recommendations for the specific situation at the hair salon. Our recommendations are based on the hierarchy of controls approach (refer to the Appendix: Occupational Exposure Limits and Health Effects). This approach groups actions by their likely effectiveness in reducing or removing hazards. In most cases, the preferred approach is to eliminate hazardous materials or processes and install engineering controls to reduce exposure or shield employees. Until such controls are in place, or if they are not effective or feasible, administrative measures and/or personal protective equipment may be needed.

Elimination and Substitution

Elimination or substitution of a toxic/hazardous process material is a highly effective means for reducing hazards. Incorporating this strategy into the design or development phase of a project, commonly referred to as "prevention through design," is most effective because it reduces the need for additional controls in the future.

- Stop using the Brazilian Blowout Acai Professional Smoothing Solution – Formaldehyde Free Formula because salon employees can be overexposed to formaldehyde.

Engineering Controls

Engineering controls reduce exposures to employees by removing the hazard from the process or placing a barrier between the hazard and the employee. Engineering controls are very effective at protecting employees without placing primary responsibility of implementation on the employee.

- Use local exhaust ventilation to reduce employee's formaldehyde exposures to below the applicable OELs if Brazilian Blowout hair smoothing product use continues despite our recommendation.

Administrative Controls

Administrative controls are management-dictated work practices and policies to reduce or prevent exposures to workplace hazards. The effectiveness of administrative changes in work practices for controlling workplace hazards is dependent on management commitment and employee acceptance. Regular monitoring and reinforcement are necessary to ensure that control policies and procedures are not circumvented in the name of convenience or production.

If the salon continues to use the Brazilian Blowout hair product it should:

- Follow the requirements listed in the OSHA formaldehyde standard [29 CFR 1910.1048]. These requirements include use of personal protective equipment, employee training, availability of eye and skin washing equipment, and employee medical surveillance.
- Conduct air sampling to further characterize employee exposures to formaldehyde.

  - If air sampling results show formaldehyde concentrations above the OSHA PEL, AL, or STEL follow the requirements as described in the OSHA formaldehyde standard. Review the OSHA hazard alert to identify different ways of reducing employee exposure to formaldehyde [OSHA 2011].

  - If sampling results show formaldehyde concentrations above the NIOSH ceiling limit or other OELs, provide employees with the appropriate NIOSH-approved respirator for use until engineering or administrative controls can be implemented to reduce formaldehyde exposures below the OELs. Respirators must be used in the context of a complete respiratory protection program in accordance with the OSHA Respiratory Protection Standard [29 CFR 1910.134].

RECOMMENDATIONS
(CONTINUED)

Personal Protective Equipment

PPE is the least effective means for controlling employee exposures. Proper use of PPE requires a comprehensive program, and calls for a high level of employee involvement and commitment to be effective. The use of PPE requires the choice of the appropriate equipment to reduce the hazard and the development of supporting programs such as training, change-out schedules, and medical assessment if needed. PPE should not be relied upon as the sole method for limiting employee exposures. Rather, PPE should be used until engineering and administrative controls can be demonstrated to be effective in limiting exposures to acceptable levels.

- Provide employees nitrile or butyl rubber gloves rather than latex gloves because of the risk of allergic reaction to natural rubber latex.

REFERENCES

Anderson S [2011]. Call for regulation of hair-smoothing products. The Associated Press. [http://safecosmetics.org/article.php?id=858]. Date accessed: September 2011.

Athavaley A [2011a]. The taming of the curl. Wall Street Journal. [http://online.wsj.com/article/SB10001424052748704461304576216470789970688.html]. Date accessed: September 2011.

Athavaley A [2011b]. Call for FDA to regulate hair straighteners. Wall Street Journal. [http://online.wsj.com/article/SB10001424052748703421204576327583570589222.html]. Date accessed: September 2011.

California OSHA [2010]. Hair smoothing products that may contain or release formaldehyde. [http://www.dir.ca.gov/dosh/HairSmoothingPageVersion1Nov182010.pdf]. Date accessed: September 2011.

CFR. Code of Federal Regulations. Washington, DC: U.S. Government Printing Office, Office of the Federal Register.

Consumer Federation of America [2011]. Consumers and hair care professionals should be cautious when using or applying "keratin-based" hair smoothing products. [http://consumerfed.org/pdfs/CIR-hair-smoother-press-release.pdf]. Date accessed: September 2011.

Dalva G [2011]. Brazilian Blowout – MSDS. Private e-mail message to Srinivas Durgam (sdurgam@cdc.gov), May 10.

EPA [2011]. EPA air toxics method – monitoring methods. [http://www.epa.gov/ttnamti1/airtox.html]. Date accessed: September 2011.

FDA [2011]. FDA receives complaints associated with the use of Brazilian Blowout. [http://www.fda.gov/Cosmetics/ProductandIngredientSafety/ProductInformation/ucm228898.htm]. Date accessed: September 2011.

Fischer MA [2007]. Scared straight. Allure the beauty expert. [http://www.allure.com/beauty-trends/how-to/2007/scared_straight]. Date accessed: September 2011.

REFERENCES
(CONTINUED)

Hayt E [2007]. Curls, splits! Ringlets, be gone! New York Times. [http://www.nytimes.com/2007/07/19/fashion/19skin1.html]. Date accessed: September 2011.

Health Canada [2011]. Several professional hair smoothing solutions contain excess levels of formaldehyde. [http://www.hc-sc.gc.ca/ahc-asc/media/advisories-avis/_2011/2011_56-eng.php]. Date accessed: September 2011.

Hollund BE, Moen BE [1998]. Chemical exposures in hairdresser salons: effect of local exhaust ventilation. Ann Occup Hyg 42(4):277–281.

Labreche F, Forest J, Trottie M, Lalonde M, Simard R [2003]. Characterization of chemical exposures in hairdressing salons. App Occup Environ Hyg 18(12):1014–1021.

Mendes A, Madureira J, Neves P, Carvalhais C, Laffon B, Teixeira JP [2011]. Chemical exposure and occupation symptoms among Portuguese hairdressers. J Tox Env Health, Part A 74(15–16):993–1000.

NIOSH [2011]. NIOSH manual of analytical methods (NMAM®). 4th ed. Schlecht PC, O'Connor PF, eds. Cincinnati, OH: U.S. Department of Health and Human Services, Centers for Disease Control and Prevention, National Institute for Occupational Safety and Health, DHHS (NIOSH) Publication 94-113 (August 1994); 1st Supplement Publication 96-135, 2nd Supplement Publication 98-119; 3rd Supplement 2003-154. [http://www.cdc.gov/niosh/docs/2003-154/]. Date accessed: September 2011.

NIST [2011]. Formaldehyde. National Institute for Standards and Technology Standard Reference Database 69: NIST Chemistry Web Book. [http://webbook.nist.gov/cgi/cbook.cgi?ID=C50000&Units=SI]. Date accessed September 2011.

Oregon OSHA [2010a]. "Keratin-based" hair smoothing products and the presence of formaldehyde. [http://www.orosha.org/pdf/Final_Hair_Smoothing_Report.pdf]. Date accessed: September 2011.

Oregon OSHA [2010b]. Oregon OSHA reiterates caution to salons using hair-smoothing products. [http://www.orosha.org/admin/newsrelease/2010/nr2010_28.pdf]. Date accessed: September 2011.

REFERENCES (CONTINUED)

OSHA [2011]. Hazard alert – hair smoothing products that could release formaldehyde. [http://www.osha.gov/SLTC/formaldehyde/hazard_alert.html]. Date accessed: September 2011.

Pristin T [2010]. A safety kink in hair relaxing. New York Times. [http://www.nytimes.com/2010/11/04/fashion/04SKIN.html]. Date accessed: September 2011.

Rabin RC [2010]. Safety: scrutiny for hair–straightening treatment. New York Times. [http://www.nytimes.com/2010/10/12/health/research/12safety.html]. Date accessed: September 2011.

The Associated Press [2011]. U.S. warns against Brazilian blowout. New York Times. [http://www.nytimes.com/2011/04/13/us/13brfs-USWARNSAGAIN_BRF.html]. Date accessed: September 2011.

Winkelman JGM, Voorwinde OK, Ottens M, Beenackers AACM, Jansen LPBM [2002]. Kinetics and chemical equilibrium of the hydration of formaldehyde. Chem Eng Sci 57(19):4067–4076.

APPENDIX: OCCUPATIONAL EXPOSURE LIMITS AND HEALTH EFFECTS

In evaluating the hazards posed by workplace exposures, NIOSH investigators use both mandatory (legally enforceable) and recommended OELs for chemical, physical, and biological agents as a guide for making recommendations. OELs have been developed by federal agencies and safety and health organizations to prevent the occurrence of adverse health effects from workplace exposures. Generally, OELs suggest levels of exposure that most employees may be exposed to for up to 10 hours per day, 40 hours per week, for a working lifetime, without experiencing adverse health effects. However, not all employees will be protected from adverse health effects even if their exposures are maintained below these levels. A small percentage may experience adverse health effects because of individual susceptibility, a preexisting medical condition, and/or a hypersensitivity (allergy). In addition, some hazardous substances may act in combination with other workplace exposures, the general environment, or with medications or personal habits of the employee to produce adverse health effects even if the occupational exposures are controlled at the level set by the exposure limit. Also, some substances can be absorbed by direct contact with the skin and mucous membranes in addition to being inhaled, which contributes to the individual's overall exposure.

Most OELs are expressed as a TWA exposure. A TWA refers to the average exposure during a normal 8- to 10-hour workday. Some chemical substances and physical agents have recommended STEL or ceiling values where adverse health effects are caused by exposures over a short period. Unless otherwise noted, the STEL is a 15-minute TWA exposure that should not be exceeded at any time during a workday, and the ceiling limit is an exposure that should not be exceeded at any time.

In the United States, OELs have been established by federal agencies, professional organizations, state and local governments, and other entities. Some OELs are legally enforceable limits, while others are recommendations. The U.S. Department of Labor OSHA PELs (29 CFR 1910 [general industry]; 29 CFR 1926 [construction industry]; and 29 CFR 1917 [maritime industry]) are legal limits enforceable in workplaces covered under the Occupational Safety and Health Act of 1970. NIOSH RELs are recommendations based on a critical review of the scientific and technical information available on a given hazard and the adequacy of methods to identify and control the hazard. NIOSH RELs can be found in the NIOSH Pocket Guide to Chemical Hazards [NIOSH 2010]. NIOSH also recommends different types of risk management practices (e.g., engineering controls, safe work practices, employee education/ training, personal protective equipment, and exposure and medical monitoring) to minimize the risk of exposure and adverse health effects from these hazards. Other OELs that are commonly used and cited in the United States include the TLVs recommended by ACGIH, a professional organization, and the WEELs recommended by the American Industrial Hygiene Association, another professional organization. The TLVs and WEELs are developed by committee members of these associations from a review of the published, peer-reviewed literature. They are not consensus standards. ACGIH TLVs are considered voluntary exposure guidelines for use by industrial hygienists and others trained in this discipline "to assist in the control of health hazards" [ACGIH 2011]. WEELs have been established for some chemicals "when no other legal or authoritative limits exist" [AIHA 2011].

Outside the United States, OELs have been established by various agencies and organizations and include both legal and recommended limits. The Institut für Arbeitsschutz der Deutschen Gesetzlichen Unfallversicherung (IFA, Institute for Occupational Safety and Health of the German Social Accident

Insurance) maintains a database of international OELs from European Union member states, Canada (Québec), Japan, Switzerland, and the United States. The database, available at http://www.dguv.de/ifa/en/gestis/limit_values/index.jsp, contains international limits for over 1,500 hazardous substances and is updated periodically.

Employers should understand that not all hazardous chemicals have specific OSHA PELs, and for some agents the legally enforceable and recommended limits may not reflect current health-based information. However, an employer is still required by OSHA to protect its employees from hazards even in the absence of a specific OSHA PEL. OSHA requires an employer to furnish employees a place of employment free from recognized hazards that cause or are likely to cause death or serious physical harm [Occupational Safety and Health Act of 1970 (Public Law 91–596, sec. 5(a)(1))]. Thus, NIOSH investigators encourage employers to make use of other OELs when making risk assessments and risk management decisions to best protect the health of their employees. NIOSH investigators also encourage the use of the traditional hierarchy of controls approach to eliminate or minimize identified workplace hazards. This includes, in order of preference, the use of (1) substitution or elimination of the hazardous agent, (2) engineering controls (e.g , local exhaust ventilation, process enclosure, dilution ventilation), (3) administrative controls (e.g., limiting time of exposure, employee training, work practice changes, medical surveillance), and (4) personal protective equipment (e.g., respiratory protection, gloves, eye protection, hearing protection). Control banding, a qualitative risk assessment and risk management tool, is a complementary approach to protecting employee health that focuses resources on exposure controls by describing how a risk needs to be managed. Information on control banding is available at http://www.cdc.gov/niosh/topics/ctrlbanding/. This approach can be applied in situations where OELs have not been established or can be used to supplement the OELs, when available.

Below we provide the OEL and a discussion of the potential health effects from exposure to formaldehyde.

Formaldehyde

Under the OSHA general industry standard for airborne exposure to formaldehyde [29 CFR 1910.1048], the PEL is 0.75 ppm for an 8-hour TWA, the AL is 0.5 ppm for an 8-hour TWA, and the STEL is 2 ppm for a 15-minute TWA. The standard requires medical surveillance for employees exposed to formaldehyde at or above the AL or STEL.

The NIOSH REL for formaldehyde is 0.016 ppm for up to an 8-hour TWA. NIOSH also has a 15-minute ceiling limit of 0.1 ppm that is not to be exceeded during a work shift [NIOSH 2010]. NIOSH recognized formaldehyde as a potential occupational carcinogen in 1981 and, following the NIOSH carcinogen policy in existence at the time, set the REL to the "lowest feasible concentration," which for formaldehyde was defined as the analytical limit of quantification of 0.016 ppm for up to 8 hours [NIOSH 1981]. Since then, experience has shown that this REL is actually not the "lowest feasible concentration" because formaldehyde in the ambient air can exceed 0.016 ppm, a fact later acknowledged by NIOSH [Lemen 1987]. Additionally, the subsequent revision of the NIOSH carcinogen policy [NIOSH 1995], combined with better exposure characterization and advances in risk assessment and management strategies, support the need for NIOSH to reassess the formaldehyde REL. This effort is in progress.

The ACGIH lists formaldehyde as a sensitizer and has a ceiling limit of 0.3 ppm [ACGIH 2011]. An ACGIH ceiling limit is an exposure that should not be exceeded at any time during the work shift.

The most commonly reported and best documented health complaints due to exposure to low concentrations of formaldehyde include irritation of the eyes, nose, and throat; nasal congestion; headaches; skin rash; and asthma. It is often difficult to attribute specific health effects to particular concentrations of formaldehyde because some people may have symptoms at levels where others may experience no symptoms. For example, irritant effects may occur in some people exposed to formaldehyde at concentrations below 0.10 ppm, but more typically irritation may not occur until exposures are at levels of 1.0 ppm or greater. However, individuals with pre-existing allergies or respiratory disease and people who have become sensitized from prior exposure may experience symptoms due to exposure to concentrations of formaldehyde between 0.05 and 0.10 ppm [NRC 1981]. Formaldehyde is also a skin sensitizer [Markowitz 2005]. In addition, the International Agency for Research on Cancer classifies formaldehyde as a human carcinogen (group 1) on the basis of associations between formaldehyde exposure and nasopharyngeal cancer and leukemia [Baan et al. 2009]. NIOSH considers formaldehyde as a potential occupational carcinogen; ACGIH lists formaldehyde as a suspected human carcinogen; and the U.S. Department of Health and Human Services lists formaldehyde as reasonably anticipated to be a human carcinogen in its 11th report on carcinogens [NIOSH 1981; ACGIH 2011; DHHS 2011].

References

ACGIH [2011]. 2011 TLVs® and BEIs®: threshold limit values for chemical substances and physical agents and biological exposure indices. Cincinnati, OH: American Conference of Governmental Industrial Hygienists.

AIHA [2011]. AIHA 2011 Emergency response planning guidelines (ERPG) & workplace environmental exposure levels (WEEL) handbook. Fairfax, VA: American Industrial Hygiene Association.

Baan R, Grosse Y, Straif K, Secretan B, El Ghissassi F, Bouvard V, Benbrahim-Tallaa L, Guha N, Freeman C, Galichet L, Cogliano V, on the behalf of the WHO International Agency for Research on Cancer Monograph Working Group [2009]. A review of human carcinogens-Part F: chemical agents and related occupations. Lancet Oncol 10(12):1143–1144.

CFR. Code of Federal Regulations. Washington, DC: U.S. Government Printing Office, Office of the Federal Register.

DHHS [2011]. Addendum to the 12th report on carcinogens. U.S. Department of Health and Human Services, National Toxicology Program. [http://ntp.niehs.nih.gov/ntp/roc/twelfth/Addendum.pdf]. Date accessed: November 2011.

Lemen RA [1987]. Official letter of February 9, 1987, from R A. Lemen, Director, Division of Standards Development and Technology Transfer, National Institute for Occupational Safety and Health, U.S. Department of Health and Human Services, Cincinnati, OH to Tom Hall, Docket Office, Department of Labor, Washington, DC.

Markowitz S [2005]. Chemicals in the plastics, synthetic textiles, and rubber industries. In: Rosenstock L, Cullen MR, Brodkin CA, Redlich CA, eds. 2nd ed. rev. Textbook of clinical occupational and environmental medicine. Philadelphia, PA: Elsevier Saunders, pp. 1008–1029.

NIOSH [1981]. Current intelligence bulletin 34 – formaldehyde: evidence of carcinogenicity. Cincinnati, OH: U.S. Department of Health and Human Services, Centers for Disease Control, National Institute for Occupational Safety and Health. DHHS (NIOSH) Publication No. 81-111 (1981, updated 1997). [http://www.cdc.gov/niosh/81111_34.html]. Date accessed: September 2011.

NIOSH [1995]. NIOSH recommended exposure limit policy. September 1995. In: NIOSH policy statements. Cincinnati, OH: U.S. Department of Health and Human Services, Centers for Disease Control and Prevention, National Institute for Occupational Safety and Health.

NIOSH [2010]. NIOSH pocket guide to chemical hazards. Cincinnati, OH: U.S. Department of Health and Human Services, Centers for Disease Control and Prevention, National Institute for Occupational Safety and Health, DHHS (NIOSH) Publication No. 2010-168c. [http://www.cdc.gov/niosh/npg/]. Date accessed: September 2011.

NRC [1981]. Formaldehyde and other aldehydes. National Research Council (National Academy Press), Washington, DC. [http://www.archive.org/stream/formaldehydeando003763mbp/formaldehydeando003763mbp_djvu.txt]. Date accessed: September 2011.

ACKNOWLEDGMENTS AND AVAILABILITY OF REPORT

The Hazard Evaluations and Technical Assistance Branch (HETAB) of the National Institute for Occupational Safety and Health (NIOSH) conducts field investigations of possible health hazards in the workplace. These investigations are conducted under the authority of Section 20(a)(6) of the Occupational Safety and Health Act of 1970, 29 U.S.C. 669(a)(6) which authorizes the Secretary of Health and Human Services, following a written request from any employer or authorized representative of employees, to determine whether any substance normally found in the place of employment has potentially toxic effects in such concentrations as used or found. HETAB also provides, upon request, technical and consultative assistance to federal, state, and local agencies; labor; industry; and other groups or individuals to control occupational health hazards and to prevent related trauma and disease.

Mention of any company or product does not constitute endorsement by NIOSH. In addition, citations to websites external to NIOSH do not constitute NIOSH endorsement of the sponsoring organizations or their programs or products. Furthermore, NIOSH is not responsible for the content of these websites. All Web addresses referenced in this document were accessible as of the publication date.

This report was prepared by Srinivas Durgam and Elena Page of HETAB, Division of Surveillance, Hazard Evaluations and Field Studies Analytical support was provided by Bureau Veritas North America. Industrial hygiene equipment and logistical support was provided by Donald Booher and Karl Feldmann. Health communication assistance was provided by Stefanie Evans. Editorial assistance was provided by Ellen Galloway. Desktop publishing was performed by Greg Hartle.

Copies of this report have been sent to employee and management representatives at the hair salon, the state health department, and the Occupational Safety and Health Administration Regional Office. This report is not copyrighted and may be freely reproduced. The report may be viewed and printed at http://www.cdc.gov/niosh/hhe/. Copies may be purchased from the National Technical Information Service at 5825 Port Royal Road, Springfield, Virginia 22161.

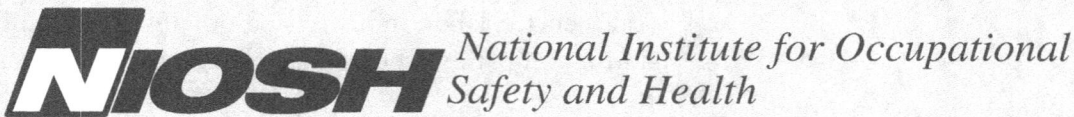

National Institute for Occupational Safety and Health

Delivering on the Nation's promise: Safety and health at work for all people through research and prevention.

To receive NIOSH documents or information about occupational safety and health topics, contact NIOSH at:

1-800-CDC-INFO (1-800-232-4636)

TTY: 1-888-232-6348

E-mail: cdcinfo@cdc.gov

or visit the NIOSH web site at: **www.cdc.gov/niosh.**

For a monthly update on news at NIOSH, subscribe to NIOSH eNews by visiting **www.cdc.gov/niosh/eNews.**

SAFER • HEALTHIER • PEOPLE™